THE
MELANATED
Milkyway
BREASTFEEDING GUIDEBOOK

THE MELANATED
Milkyway
BREASTFEEDING GUIDEBOOK

SHAQUANNA

Only Black Stars in the Sky
Thomasville, NC

THE MELANATED MILKYWAY BREASTFEEDING GUIDEBOOK
The author has provided this material for the readers' information.
It is not intended to substitute the medical expertise and
advice of a healthcare provider. Readers are encouraged to
discuss any decisions about treatment or care with a licensed
healthcare provider. The mention of any product, service, or
therapy is not an endorsement by the author or publisher.

THE MELANATED MILKYWAY BREASTFEEDING GUIDEBOOK
Copyright © 2020 Shaquanna Thomas

Paperback ISBN-13: 978-0-578-73634-1

Only Black Stars in the Sky
Thomasville, NC

Printed in the United States of America
First Edition September 2020

Cover Design: Make Your Mark Publishing Solutions
Design: Make Your Mark Publishing Solutions
Editing: Make Your Mark Publishing Solutions

Contents

Acknowledgements

I would like to give a million thanks to the women who inspire me every day, from my kindred to my social media associates. The network of support, both physical and virtual, has been a reliable lifeline for me through the years.

Thank you to all the birth workers and educators who support melanated families on their transition into parenthood. You are valuable.

I extend much gratitude to my husband, who is my number one supporter. You were my alpha reader and reviewer and continue to be an amazing team leader. Your dynamic presence in my life contributes greatly to me reaching my breastfeeding goals and striving for all of my dreams.

Introduction

I've heard it all: "Some women just can't breastfeed." "I've tried to breastfeed, but my milk never came in." "My baby was jaundice, so I had to supplement with formula." All of these statements, and more, are common, but for the vast majority of women, these words are simply untrue. These are myths perpetuated by formula companies and spread through fear-based tactics. Telling a mom her child will starve if she doesn't supplement with formula is a good way to keep a loyal customer. Fear is primal, but so is breastfeeding. By centering education as the primary resource for breastfeeding mothers, my goal is to remove the fear and replace it with awareness.

The fact is, both mom and baby are at an increased risk of illnesses when the breastfeeding relationship is severed or not initiated. The myths associated with breastfeeding cause more harm among the Black/Indigenous communities because of our complex history of miseducation from doctors, wet nursing, and the blatant push of artificial foods/formulas over breast-milk. Our mothers lack the community and professional and generational support to sustain breastfeeding throughout the first year of their babies' lives. The lack of support often results in moms quitting before they've reached their intended goal, with the most common complaints being painful latching, returning to work, and low milk supply. These are multi-faceted variables and intersectional issues, which must be handled accordingly, by someone who is culturally competent. That is why I wrote this guidebook.

In this book, you will learn the basics of breastfeeding, how to recognize a potential problem, and when to seek professional help for your issues. Having a fundamental understanding of breastfeeding will create an atmosphere of confidence and security for families pursuing the journey. When I first became a mother, I was only able to breastfeed my child for four months. It broke my heart to not have the support or education to reach my one-year goal. After many years of research, I was able to develop the skills I needed to successfully breastfeed premature twins until their second birthday. I never once had to use formula as a supplement, even when they were in the hospital being fed via feeding tubes.

If you or someone you love has a desire to breast-feed, *The Melanated Milkyway* is a useful gift to receive or give. I wrote this book as a peer-to-peer resource, with no judgement. This is a conversation between two moms—you and me—on how to navigate the concerns that come up when breastfeeding. This breastfeeding guidebook is perfectly structured to be both a manual and a tool. It will guide you on your journey while also providing you with the resources you need to meet your breastfeeding goals. This book, however, is not a replacement for a lactation professional like an IBCLC or CLC. Lactation professionals are still an important part of breastfeeding education and were integral in my own success, which is why I began studying to become one.

Breastfeeding is natural, but natural does not mean easy. Here, you have a partner, and you'll find everything you need to know so you may breastfeed with confidence.

CHAPTER 1

❖ ✦ ❖

Breastfeeding Rules

Some of these may seem obvious—others, not so much. These "rules" are in keeping with breastfeeding best practices based on relevant research.

1. **No pumping in the first six weeks.** Hand-expressing is a better option. In the first week following their birth, breastfed babies can lose about seven to ten percent of their birth weight. Weight loss in the first week is not a reason to pump or supplement with formula. Pumping in the first six weeks is not recommended because doing so can create an oversupply. During this

time, your baby will be regulating your supply by nursing frequently. If you begin to pump in addition to nursing, your body will make milk to accommodate for the pump as if it were another baby. Hand-express for comfort and relief, but do not try to "empty" the breast.

2. **Never pump and dump.** Milk can always be used for something else. Pumping and dumping is an outdated concept. Your milk is liquid gold and can be used in a variety of ways, such as in milk baths, lotions for the body, relief for cracked nipples, and more.

3. **Don't detox or start a fast/diet**. Doing any of these can cause impurities in your milk. See Chapter 9.

4. **Don't skip feedings.** Too many missed feedings can reduce milk production. Do not skip feedings. Skipping feedings can result in a lower milk supply. Milk is supply and demand. Your body will only continue making enough milk if you remove it from your breast every two to three hours. Even at night, you should nurse (or pump, if exclusively pumping or if baby is in the neonatal intensive care unit [NICU]).

5. **Colostrum is milk.** Baby will only need a few drops in the first few days. Colostrum is a thick, yellow/gold milk that will be your baby's first meal. This is the first milk your baby will receive from you, and it will be all they need in those first few days. Do not feel pressured to supplement with formula. If you have to pump due to an emergency, be aware that colostrum is very thick and cannot be removed from the breasts easily. A suckling baby has an easier time removing the liquid gold than a pump. Hand-expressing a few drops for your baby will be enough until you are able to latch or until your transitional milk appears two to four days postpartum.

6. **Your milk is enough.** Newborns feed frequently to regulate your supply.

7. **Skin-to-skin contact, a.k.a kangaroo care, is essential to your journey.** Skin-to-skin contact is when your bare skin comes in contact with your naked or partially dressed newborn. This practice aids in regulating their body temperature and blood sugar levels and promotes milk production. I highly recommend babywearing for easy, hands-free skin-to-skin contact.

Babywearing is the process of carrying a baby in a sling or another carrier, also referred to as kangaroo care. If you have multiples, you can carry two babies at a time. You may need assistance if you have more than two newborns.

8. **A good latch won't hurt.** Discomfort is normal. Tear-worthy pain is not. When first learning how to breastfeed, your nipples can be tender. This can cause discomfort and pain during the latching process. The pain should only last a few seconds and should be mild to moderate. If the pain lasts longer than that or is more severe, it is likely an improper latch. See Chapter 2 to read more about a proper latch.

9. **Baby can't be overfed at the breast.** Spit-up is normal. Projectile vomit is not. Babies cannot be overfed at the breasts because they are in control of the milk flow and their intake. Babies can, however, be overfed via a bottle. Spit-up is not a sign that baby is being overfed. In most cases, it's perfectly normal. The baby is brand new, and their body has to learn how to digest breastmilk, which often triggers a bit of spit-up. Projectile vomit, on the other hand, is a sign of something being potentially wrong. Speak to a healthcare

professional as soon as possible if your baby is projectile vomiting.

10. **Breastfeeding is natural**, but it also requires dedication and education. Breastfeeding is as natural as giving birth, but it will require time and dedication to get right. Some women never experience any problems when breastfeeding, while others have a different story to tell. Take classes, read books, join support groups, speak to a lactation consultant, get resources from the government's Women, Infants, and Children (WIC) program, and always ask for help. Natural does not mean easy.

There are exceptions to every rule. Some women will need to pump if they decide to return to work before six weeks or due to an emergency. Other women will choose to exclusively pump. However, pumping is not required to have a successful breastfeeding journey. Always seek professional help if you feel your baby may not be getting enough milk.

CHAPTER 2

✦ ◆ ✦

The Golden Hour

The first hour following birth is the most important time, as a baby's instinct to breastfeed peaks about twenty to thirty minutes after they are born, regardless of if the birth was vaginal or cesarean. These first crucial moments are not the time for healthcare professionals to take your baby to have measurements done, the first bath (which is not needed, as babies are not born dirty), or any other non-emergency procedures can wait until after the golden hour has passed.

During this time, the baby will learn how to latch properly. Here are a few tips to help you when assisting your little one:

1. Align your baby's nose with your nipple.
2. Make sure your and your baby's tummies are touching. Use a pillow if you had a cesarean birth. (Ask for a tummy binder if you had surgery.)
3. Make sure baby's arms are spread like a hug, with one on top of the breast and the other beneath.
4. Make sure your hand is supporting, not pushing, the back of your baby's head.
5. Wait until their mouth is opened wide, like a yawn, before bringing them to the nipple. You can gently squeeze or sandwich the areola to make the area smaller for baby to get a deeper latch.
6. Bring your baby up to the breast. Do not lean down to meet the baby.
7. Baby's lips should be flanged like a fish against the breast.
8. Be sure you are not hunching your shoulders or leaning forward. Over time, this can cause a sore back and neck.
9. If baby is latched improperly, unlatch them by putting a finger in the side of their mouth along the cheek to break the latch. An improper latch will be painful or uncomfortable for more than a few seconds.

If you have inverted nipples, stimulate them by rubbing and gently pulling on them to cause them to become slightly erect. Inverted nipples appear flat against the areola or go inward. This is not an indication that a woman cannot breastfeed. Pumping for about two to three minutes can also aid in pulling the nipple out and can make it easier for baby to latch. There is no need to pump long enough to express milk because pumping in the first six weeks can cause an oversupply and other breast-related issues. To avoid nipple confusion, it is best to not introduce a bottle or pacifier for the first six weeks or until breastfeeding has been properly established.

Other benefits of the golden hour include increased bonding between mom and baby, increased chances for a successful breastfeeding relationship, calmer moods and less stress for mom and baby, delayed cord clamping, and a decreased risk of infection. The golden hour should be spent doing skin-to-skin contact with your newborn. This is also a good time to rub the vernix, the white, creamy substance coating your baby after they are born, into their skin. The amino acids work to protect your baby against harmful bacteria, such as B Streptococcus and E. coli. It also helps control body temperature, keeps baby's skin moisturized and soft, and produces that new baby smell that promotes bonding between mother and child. Since the vernix does not fully absorb into the skin for five to six days, it is best to delay the first bath until then.

CHAPTER 3

✦ ◆ ✦

Well-Fed Babies and Diaper Output

Is my baby gaining weight? How is their diaper output? The answer to these two questions is what determines if your baby is getting enough milk. During the first week after birth, babies usually have one wet diaper per each numbered day—one soiled diaper on day one, two on day two, and so on. After your mature milk comes in, expect five to seven wet diapers and three to four poop diapers a day. You can also expect to nurse ten to twelve times in a twenty-four-hour period. In the first week following their birth, breastfed babies will lose roughly seven to ten percent of their birth weight. Do not count this loss when determining if your baby is gaining weight.

After their initial weight loss, your baby should gain around six ounces a week. Wet diapers should be pale yellow to clear in color. If the diapers are darker in color after the first few days, check with your healthcare professional to ensure your baby is getting enough milk. Orange urine can be a sign of dehydration. Baby stools or poop should be mustard yellow and seedy after the first few days.

Watch the baby, not the clock. Babies nurse for different reasons, including comfort, thirst, or hunger. They will also nurse for different amounts of time. Do not remove the baby from your breast if you *think* they are done eating or if they have been on the breast "too long." Allow your baby to come off the breast on their own, then offer the other side. Baby may refuse or accept the second breast.

Cluster feeding is when a baby nurses constantly or frequently for several hours or days. This can make you feel like you are doing something wrong or that your milk is not enough. Despite those feelings, you must trust you are enough. Your breasts are never empty; as long as baby is nursing, milk is being made. Cluster feeding is a way for your baby to signal your body to make more milk. These, along with growth spurts, usually happen around the first few days after birth, seven to ten days after birth, two to three weeks postpartum, and four to six weeks postpartum. Keep these timelines in mind if you begin to have any concerns.

Feed your baby at the first sign of hunger. Signs of hunger include:

- Putting their hands to their face and mouth
- Making sucking sounds
- Turning their heads and opening their mouth, a.k.a. rooting
- Getting in a breastfeeding position

Do not wait until after your baby has started to be noticeably angry and/or crying to feed them. A frustrated baby has a hard time latching and will get more agitated at the breast. If your baby is already crying, try to soothe them by standing up, gently rocking, and making soft cooing sounds.

Low Supply

Very few women (less than two percent) have a true issue with low supply. The following *does not* indicate a low supply:

- Soft breasts
- Breasts that are no longer engorged

- Low pump output
- Baby being fussy at the breast
- Breasts no longer (or never) leaking
- Baby waking frequently to eat
- Baby taking expressed breastmilk or formula after a feeding (top-up trap)
- Baby nursing too long or not long enough (watch the baby, not the clock)
- Family/friends saying your baby isn't full

The breasts are not meant to remain hard and engorged as they were in the first days and weeks after giving birth. Soft breasts are normal and do not indicate that your milk supply has decreased. The volume of blood that was needed to jumpstart breastfeeding in those first days postpartum is no longer necessary, which allows your breasts to become softer over time and reduce engorgement. This is also why you may not leak anymore.

The pump cannot determine how much milk has been produced by the body. Not responding to the pump or pumping very little is not a sign that the milk is not there at all. Some women simply do not respond well to the pump but will have better luck with hand-expressing their milk. If your baby is waking to eat frequently, becoming fussy at the breast, or is nursing too long or too little, understand that these are not out of the realm of normal behaviors. Babies nurse for a variety of reasons, food and comfort being among them. Keep your baby close, watch for signs of hunger, and nurse on demand. Do not be tempted to give your baby extra milk in a bottle or by any other method other than your breast, as this can cause overfeeding and begin the top-up trap.

The top-up trap is when you doubt your ability to nurse your child from the breast, so a supplemental feeding is given. This, in turn, causes the baby to turn away from the breast and latch less, which signals the body to produce less milk due to a lack of stimulation and milk removal, thus causing you to doubt your ability to breastfeed again. If anyone is filling your head with doubts, please seek out a professional and a peer group. Having support is paramount to your success.

There are several reasons you could be experiencing a low milk supply. Some of the most common causes for a low milk supply include:

- Taking oral hormonal birth control
- Poor nipple latching, tongue tie, or lip tie
- Retained placenta fragments
- Not positioning your baby correctly during feedings
- Postpartum hemorrhages
- Previous breast reduction surgery or trauma (not all but a few)

- Medications, such as antihistamines and decongestants
- Supplementing with a bottle without expressing breastmilk (skipping feedings)
- Chronic conditions, such as diabetes, thyroid diseases, and polycystic ovary syndrome (PCOS)
- Menstrual cycle

If any of these resonate with you and you would still like to continue breastfeeding, speak to your healthcare professional about alternatives, make an appointment with a breastfeeding specialist, and do some research yourself about the different paths you can take to reach your breastfeeding goals without putting your health at risk.

Some moms may require milk donations from other nursing mothers. I discuss milk donations more in Chapter 8.

CHAPTER 4

✦ ◆ ✦

Troubleshooting Breastfeeding Worries

Cracked Nipples

Cracked nipples can result from an improper latch, dry skin, or skin irritation by clothing, damp milk pads, or chemicals. Correcting the issue that caused the cracked nipples is the most efficient way to prevent your nipples from becoming damaged in the future. One of the best remedies for this is your own breastmilk. Coconut oil, olive oil, and certain breastfeeding-safe topical ointments can also help keep your nipples and areolas moisturized to better prevent breaks and skin abrasions. It's also important to keep your nipples exposed to air to promote effective healing.

Clogged Ducts

Examine your breasts for a nipple pore or milk blister. Has your milk slowed down in one breast? Is one breast particularly swollen or tender? Is there pain in one area? Are their small lumps or hard areas? If you answered yes to any of these questions, you may have a clogged duct.

How to Relieve a Clogged/Plugged Milk Duct

- Combing your breast from the armpit to the areola can dislodge a clog. Yes, you read that correctly.
- A hot compress or shower can relieve pressure and milk from the tender area. An herbal compress can also be an effective method of removing a clog. Be careful not to damage or burn your skin.
- Let gravity work with you by hovering safely over your baby or breast pump to help move the clog down. You can also dangle over a bowl of warm water and Epsom salt.
- Regular breast massages can support your overall breast health. While trying to remove a clog, you want to massage the clogged area more

frequently in combination with hand expression or pumping.

- Having your partner provide light to moderate suckling in the direction of the clog can be very beneficial in moving the clog. Your baby may not provide enough force and can become frustrated at the reduced milk flow, so ask your partner for help to release a clogged duct.

Do not let a clog "go away on its own" because this can lead to lower milk production, pain, or even mastitis, an infection and inflammation of the breast that requires antibiotics.

Thrush

Thrush is a common type of yeast infection caused by a fungus called candida. Itchy or burning nipples is the most common symptom of nipple thrush. Your nipples and areola may also look pale or you may form red, itchy rashes. Thrush typically appears as white or yellow irregularly shaped patches or sores that coat your baby's gums and tongue, along with the sides and roof of the mouth. There are many home remedies available to treat thrush, including:

- Probiotics
- Saltwater rinse

- Sugar-free yogurt
- Direct sunlight
- Baking soda rinse
- Gentian violet (fungicidal violet dye)
- Over-the-counter antifungal creams

If the thrush is severe, your healthcare provider may prescribe an antifungal medicine. Treat your nipples and breasts, along with your baby, to prevent recontamination. If you are using bottles, use special care and cleaning to avoid reintroducing the infection to your baby and yourself.

Mastitis

Mastitis is an inflammation of breast tissue that sometimes involves an infection. The inflammation results in breast pain, swelling, warmth, and redness. You might also have a fever and chills. It can be treated with prescription antibiotics, colloidal silver (more information is available through the bibliography), and garlic.

You can prevent mastitis by properly and thoroughly removing milk from the breast. If you have an oversupply, this may become more difficult and time consuming.

- Express milk every two to three hours. Do not try to stretch out your nursing/pumping sessions.
- Do not allow your breasts to become engorged often after your milk has regulated (six to eight weeks postpartum).
- Always remove clogged ducts.
- Wear a fitted bra (if you need it) and loose-fitting clothes.
- Avoid prolonged use of nipple ointments, creams, and pads (synthetic or cloth).
- Wash your hands after changing the baby.

Baby Bonding and Special Circumstances

Breastfeeding can cause you to feel happy, hungry, thirsty, and like a goddess, but you can also feel overwhelmed, unappreciated, and touched out. These are all normal feelings. Having a tiny body feeding off of you can cause many emotions to fill your body and mind. Naturally, breastfeeding releases endorphins and the "love hormone" oxytocin, which makes you feel happy and bonded with your baby. If you don't feel happy and bonded immediately, that is also normal. There is no right way to feel. However, if you are having invading memories or thoughts, negative feelings associated with nursing or pumping, extreme exhaustion and fatigue, or unpleasant emotions while being touched by your baby, you could be experiencing postpartum depression. Talk to your healthcare provider, an international board-certified lactation consultant (IBCLC), a therapist, or a birth and lactation educator who is equipped to assist you. Do not suffer in silence.

Talking to someone about mental health can be scary. You could be experiencing a fear of judgement, a fear of being seen as a bad parent, or a fear of your child being removed from your care and home. I get it, and these are all valid concerns that keep people from seeking help. One way to handle this is to be aware of the language you are using to describe your symptoms. The next is to be cognizant of who you are asking for help. A doula or traditional (not medical) midwife may be more compassionate, helpful, and understanding of what you are going through. Finally, find a local or online support group. You are not alone.

Milk Aversion

Breastfeeding or milk aversion is not uncommon among women who are breastfeeding multiples, pregnant while nursing, or are tandem nursing an infant and a toddler. Regardless of your situation, there may come a time when you prefer not to have a little one attached to your body for any moment of time, yet you muscle through anyway. Consider the following to determine what may be affecting your mood:

- Are you sleeping enough?
- Are you eating enough?
- Are you following a self-care routine?
- Have you had any alone time?
- Are you getting enough sunlight?
- Are you getting enough fresh air?
- Have you talked to another adult today?
- Is your baby cluster feeding?

Once you have gone through and, hopefully, identified the cause of your discomfort, you may be able to remedy the situation. When in doubt, eat some dark chocolate. The magnesium can help you feel relaxed, while the serotonin and endorphins can improve your overall mood. Eating dark chocolate with higher percentages will provide the best benefits.

If you experience sadness that goes away after thirty seconds to two minutes during or right before milk letdown, you could be experiencing dysphoric milk ejection reflex, or D-MER. D-MER is a condition affecting lactating women that is characterized by abrupt dysphoria that occurs just before milk release and continues no more than a few minutes. D-MER is more than an aversion to breastfeeding or being touched. It is a hormonal response to milk letdown, and a mother (like you or someone you love) cannot talk themselves out of it. Professional help and intervention are required for proper treatment.

Menses

Periods, or the time right before them, can cause a reduction in your supply. Calcium and magnesium supplements (500 to 1,000 mg) can help lessen the effects of your period. Eating pineapple, dark chocolate, and red raspberry leaf (tea or tincture) are natural ways to prevent or "treat" the symptoms of your period and can help manage your supply, as they are all rich in calcium, magnesium, and iron and easily accessible. Irish sea moss is another home remedy that moms love. The sea moss can be made into a capsule or gel and added to soups, smoothies, oatmeal, and more.

CHAPTER 5

Myths, Negative Associations, and Generational Trauma

Wet Nursing

A wet nurse is a woman who breastfeeds and cares for another's child. Wet nurses are employed if the mother is unable or elects not to nurse the child herself. Wet-nursed children may be known as "milk siblings," and in some cultures, the families are linked by a special relationship of milk kinship.

We cannot have a conversation about breastfeeding and the culture surrounding it without discussing chattel slavery and indentured servitude in the Americas. Before the slavery era, breastfeeding was a socially accepted behavior. Providing babies with a mother's milk was not a question but an obvious response to giving birth. There is a documented history of black and brown bodies being used to nurse white babies, while Black babies were left hungry or to be fed by another member of the group. This is/was heartbreaking and caused a ripple of generational backlash and trauma, the effects of which still echo throughout hospitals and epicenters of Black womanhood.

Wet nursing, or breastfeeding a baby that was not your own, was essential to group survival. Some mothers were not able to breastfeed because of an illness, separation from their baby, low milk production, or death. Throughout history, donated milk or wet nursing has always been a part of breastfeeding culture. Within the Black and Indigenous communities, wet nursing is still seen as a leftover of slavery. Because of this negative association, well-meaning mothers, grandmothers, and aunties discourage younger generations of women in their families from ever trying to breastfeed their own children.

Wet nursing did not start or stop with slavery. Late nineteenth and early twentieth century physicians used wet nursing as a means to stop the deaths of the infants who came through the hospital doors. Both private institutions and wealthy families hired wet nurses as a means to adequately feed their own babies, while the women who worked for them were told to leave their infants in the care of someone else. The same artificial foods (formula and milk) the wealthy avoided by hiring wet nurses were given to the infants of the women they employed, and roughly ninety percent of those infants died. You could draw serious comparisons to *The Handmaid's Tale* and similar stories. This has left an understandably horrible stain on breastfeeding for the generations of women who had to endure such abuse.

What does that mean for the modern Black and Indigenous women who desire to breastfeed their own children? It means breaking generational curses and going against long-held familial and cultural beliefs. It means self-education and reflection are a requirement for breastfeeding unbothered and confidently. Hospital staff, doctors, nurses, family, coworkers, strangers, and your partner can all pressure you to formula-feed for their convenience, personal beliefs, or just because they don't want to see you doing what they never did for themselves and their children. That will not be your problem. Their issues are deeply rooted; however, they are their own.

A Brief History of Formula

Formula was never considered to be an adequate substitute for human breastmilk. Never. The concoction was entirely or primarily made of cow's milk, which is not suitable for an infant other than a calf. Doctors have always agreed (until recently and we will discuss this, too) that breastmilk should be the only food source for an infant.

Joseph DeLee, known as the "father of modern obstetrics," was a Chicago doctor who was quoted in 1903 saying, "Without mother's milk, it is almost impossible to raise a premature infant—certainly to be a healthy one." Artificial feedings were troublesome and not considered sufficient for infant feedings. Families who could afford a wet nurse servant paid for one, while others saw their infants become malnourished if they refused the nursing from the women whom they deemed as beneath them.

The formulation of artificial milk was more for money and exploitation of the poor than it was for the betterment of infants and the mothers who needed to substitute the feedings. Formula has, and continues to, undermine breastmilk, especially in poor countries. Jumping forward to the 1980s, we saw undeniable proof that formula companies' marketing was unethical and deliberate in their attempt to stop mothers from their natural instinct to nurse their newborn for the sake of money.

That year, 1981, was significant because it coincided with the peak of a scandal that rocked Nestle. In 1974, a bombshell report called "The Baby Killer," published by the U.K. charity War on Want, accused the company of introducing formula to impoverished countries that it knew couldn't use the products properly, just to turn a profit.

The company's aggressive marketing in poor regions came at a time when sales were declining in the U.S. The company's shrewd marketing scheme included sending in sales representatives dressed in nurse uniforms to hospitals to give away samples and urge mothers to give up breastfeeding.

The scandal led to an international boycott against Nestle beginning in 1977 that lasted until 1984, when the company agreed to abide by the WHO's guidelines on marketing. (The company faced another boycott several years later when it resumed participating in banned marketing practices.)

— Eleanor Goldberg, Business
Reporter, HuffPost

The World Health Organization (WHO) wrote a detailed instructive for formula companies known as the International Code of Marketing of Breast-Milk Substitutes (the Code) that outlined how they were allowed to market. The USA was the only country to not adopt this code into law, and the results of that speak for themselves. Eight hundred thousand babies die every year due to lack of breastmilk. Issues like malnourishment, diarrhea, and respiratory issues could be resolved by exclusively breastfeeding for six months. Nestle was boycotted on an international level on multiple occasions spanning many years due to their use of banned marketing practices.

Myths

1. **Breastfeeding will make my baby clingy or spoiled.** All babies are clingy. Someone who just spent their entire life in utero will come out to the world small and dependent on their caregivers. No exception. Breastfeeding will not make this worse. Keeping babies close is better for

their overall brain development, the regulation of their body temperature, and their blood sugar levels; plus, it promotes skin-to-skin contact, which is important for milk production.

2. **Breastfeeding is only beneficial for six months.** Breastfeeding remains beneficial for years for both mom and baby. Breastfeeding longer than a year can lower your risk of certain types of cancers, like breast cancer, and offers lifelong immunity-boosting properties to the baby. Breastfeeding will also lower the risk of SIDS and reduce the baby's risks of infection and childhood obesity.

3. **If my baby eats too long, it means they are not getting full.** Breastmilk is easily digested, and at times, you will find that your little one poops while you are feeding. This is normal. This is also why they eat so frequently. Feeding your baby often will help regulate your supply and stimulate milk production.

4. **A full baby will sleep longer.** This is a commonly held myth among many families; however, it is not true. Babies are biologically designed to wake every few hours. Doing so lowers their chances of dying from SIDS. Breastmilk is

filling yet easily digested. Nursing on demand will ensure baby gets exactly what they need when they need it. Do not be tempted to add anything to your baby's breastmilk to make them sleep longer. Cereal is a popular additive but should never be added to a bottle, as it is a choking hazard. Babies younger than six months should not be fed any foods other than breastmilk or formula under any circumstances.

5. **Baby will use me as a pacifier.** Pacifiers are artificial nipples created to simulate the sensation of suckling at the breast. If you give a baby a pacifier in place of your breast, you could be inadvertently missing a feeding. You are the natural source of comfort and food for your little one.

6. **No one will watch my baby for me to work or go to school.** If/when you need to return to work or school, your baby will adjust. Introduce your baby to their caregiver while you are still around and allow them to feed the baby. Bottles, spoons, cups, syringes (not needles), droppers, and other tools can be used to feed your baby your expressed milk. If you are still in the house, your baby may refuse to be fed by someone else. It is not uncommon for babies to begin a hunger

strike and refuse the bottle altogether. If this happens, try not to worry, as your baby will make up for the missed feedings during your time together.

7. **Breastfeeding will make my breasts sag.** Genetics, hormones, age, weight, pregnancy, and wearing a bra are what will determine if your breasts sag, not breastfeeding. There is no way to prevent sagging, but you can promote healthier breasts and muscles by working out, going braless, keeping the breasts moisturized, practicing good posture, and receiving regular breast massages.

8. **I will have to pump to know how much my baby is getting.** Pumping is only required if you are going to be away from your baby long enough to miss one or more feedings. As long as the baby is producing enough wet/soiled diapers, they are getting enough milk.

Note: After four to six weeks postpartum, your exclusively breastfed baby can safely go two weeks without pooping. This is not an indication that something is wrong. Breastmilk is the perfect food and produces little waste.

CHAPTER 6

◆ ◆ ◆

Preemies, Ties, Multiples, and Tandem

Preemies come with unique needs based on the length of gestation and health concerns, but breastfeeding is still the best food for them. If they have a feeding tube, breastmilk can be put inside it instead of formula. Ask for a hospital-grade pump and express your milk while your baby is in the NICU. Wipe your baby's saliva onto your areola and nipple. This will send signals to your body about the kind of milk you need to produce to better aid your baby's growth and health. This happens because breastmilk is a living organism.

Doctors may try to push you to use formula for a variety of reasons, and the one I most commonly hear and have experienced firsthand is weight gain. Yes, formula has a few more calories than breastmilk; however, that does not make it the ideal food for your little one. Your breastmilk is enough and does not require formula or human milk fortifier (HMF) made from cow's milk to be "better" or more calorically dense. Big does not always mean healthy.

Human milk is easier for infants to digest than formula and does not expose their immature intestinal lining to the proteins from cow's milk that are found in infant formulas. Premature babies who are breastfed are less likely to develop intestinal infections than babies who are fed formula. No other milk or food source compares to the nourishing benefits of breastmilk, as it contains immunologic agents and other compounds that protect against viruses, bacteria, and parasites. If HMF is needed, I recommend asking for breastmilk donations from another mother as the choice supplement. It's best to get milk from the hospital or a milk bank, as these milks have been properly screened.

"Improving the Use of Human Milk During and After the NICU Stay" is a medical research article about the benefits of breastfeeding premature infants while in the NICU and once they go home. The writers of the article support colostrum as the first food for premature infants, avoiding formula during the stage of colostrum feedings, and following the colostrum feedings with mature breastmilk after three to four days postpartum.

I am not a doctor nor a medical professional. This is peer-to-peer, mother-to-mother talk in hopes I can be helpful and encouraging. If you feel like this information does not fit the needs of you and your family, you are free to make any decision you need to based on your assessment of your situation. Always consult an IBCLC or breastfeeding specialist to answer questions about your individual situation.

Here is a list of things you can do to support weight gain in your preemie:

- Massage your baby with organic coconut oil multiple times a day. This is effective because the oil will absorb into their skin. The layer of oil will also help trap heat inside of their body and prevent water loss. Both will help support a healthy weight gain.

- Skin-to-skin contact helps regulate their body temperature and stimulates milk production. It will also keep your baby calm. The more time your baby spends sleeping and not agitated, the better.

- Feed your baby on a schedule. It is important your baby eats every two to three hours like clockwork. If your baby is hungry before their scheduled feeding time, talk to the nurses and doctors about adjusting the time. Your baby should not be left to cry just because the nurses don't want to disrupt the schedule.

Tongue and Lip Ties

Tongue and lip ties are conditions that restrict the range of motion of a baby's tongue or lip. This can make it next to impossible to get a good latch and, therefore, can make you feel as if you are unable to breastfeed. This is not true. While this condition will present more challenges for you, it does not have to derail your entire journey.

Signs of a tongue or lip tie include:

- Shallow latch
- Falling off the breast
- "Clicking noises" (indicating the loss of suction and intake of air)
- Nipple and breast pain (including plugged ducts and mastitis)
- Minimal weight gain

If you suspect a tie, have your baby examined by an IBCLC, a pediatrician/pediatric dentist knowledgeable in breastfeeding, or an ear, nose, and throat specialist. Both tongue and lip ties can be treated with surgery.

Tandem Nursing and Multiples

Breastfeeding multiples is time consuming. You have the option to nurse in tandem (to free up some time) or feed each baby separately. If you are dealing with low-birth-weight babies, you may have an easier time latching and feeding them separately. As they get older and gain more weight, the feedings should become easier, and nursing in tandem will be possible if it wasn't previously. Breastfeeding pillows and wedges are a great support.

Nursing a newborn and an older baby is also doable and quite common. This is what is commonly thought of when discussing tandem nursing. The older child may start eating more often or may stop taking the breast altogether. Your body will produce milk that is appropriate for your little ones, no matter what, and the benefits of breastfeeding are extended to the older child as long as they desire the milk.

CHAPTER 7

✦ ◆ ✦

Pumping Resource and FAQs

Being away from baby is hard, and none of us want to leave before we have to. Nevertheless, some women will eventually need to return to work or school. This is a guide to help you achieve your breastfeeding goal.

Rules for Pumping

- Do not pump longer than twenty consecutive minutes. Pumping longer could damage the breast tissue.
- Do not reheat breastmilk in the microwave. This can lead to hotspots and can cause serious burns

to your baby's mouth and throat. Use a bowl of hot water to thaw frozen milk. Double bag your breastmilk when thawing to prevent leaks.

- Do not mix warm breastmilk with frozen breastmilk.
- Do not refreeze breastmilk after it has been thawed.
- Do not add anything to your breastmilk.
- Always rotate your breastmilk, keeping the oldest in the front to be used first.
- Always keep your breasts (areola and nipples) moisturized and oiled before pumping and well-ventilated/dried after pumping.
- What you pump is not an indication of your output. The pump is not as effective at removing milk as a baby.
- Use flanges, or shields, that fit. If a flange does not fit properly, your milk output can be reduced and damage to your breasts can occur.

FAQs

Will I need a breastmilk stash to go back to work/school?

Yes and no. You do not need a Pinterest-level freezer stash. A freezer full of milk is not needed to have a successful breastfeeding journey. What you will need is a day's worth of milk and a few extra ounces for emergencies. A general rule is to have one to one-and-a-half ounces of breastmilk for every hour you will be away. Include your commute time when making your calculations.

Ex: School is three hours long, with a fifteen-minute break and thirty minutes of commute time each way.

Three hours + two thirty-minute commutes + a fifteen-minute break = four hours and fifteen minutes away from baby.

If you round up to four-and-a-half hours to account for traffic or emergencies, baby will need four-and-a-half to six-and-three-quarter ounces of breastmilk that day.

You will be able to get this amount by pumping leftovers (the remaining milk after baby has been fed via breast), catching milk from the unused breast during a feeding, and pumping/hand-expressing while baby is napping.

You will need to pump or feed before you leave the house and pump during work/school two to three hours after your last session. If you need more time on your break to pump, discuss with your human resources team or school administration ahead of time. Document everything via email.

To maintain a healthy milk supply, you must pump every two to three hours you are away from baby, including commute time. If you find the commute is the only time you have to pump, you should invest in hands-free pumping devices, like Freemie cups. The silicone suction-style pump could also work for you, as long as you have a secure bra or an attachment that will not drop a full pump once the suction loosens. The phrase, "Don't cry over spilt milk" does not apply to a breastfeeding woman, so be very careful with the devices you use to collect your milk.

Remember to always reset your pump back to the lowest speed and pressure when you turn it off. Accidental injuries to your nipple can occur if your pump is set too high. Speed and pressure could cause a minor tear or a severe one across your nipple and areola if one is not careful. I have personally made this mistake and know firsthand the pain that results from forgetting to do so.

Where should I pump when I am out?

Pump where you are comfortable. If you are comfortable sitting on the floor or on a bench at the store, go for it. You can pump at a food court, in a restaurant, or anywhere you are comfortable or otherwise allowed to be. Ask for a nursing station at work or school; you may be surprised to find there is one located in the building. Even if they don't have one, your inquiry could get them thinking about one. Your workplace legally cannot make you pump in the bathroom, the break room, your car, or anywhere else that isn't shielded from view or accessible to you when you need it. You have the right to a private room. The Federal Break Time for Nursing Mothers law requires employers covered by the Fair Labor Standards Act (FLSA) to provide basic accommodations for breastfeeding mothers at work. These accommodations include time for women to express milk in a private space that is not a bathroom each time they need to pump.

Talk to your HR department about where you will be pumping *before* you go back to work. Send emails to keep a record of the exchanges, and CC all relevant management. Examine the area beforehand and make sure you won't need to schedule times, use a special pass/key, or share the room with another woman. None of these are issues, but you don't want to surprise another mom by walking in on her or not be able to get into a locked room because you don't have a code/key.

Where can I store my expressed milk?

Bring a cooler bag with you and keep your pump and expressed milk in the bag. Breastmilk can survive inside a cooler with just an ice block for a full day. Refrigerate or freeze your milk when you get home. Do not leave your milk in the community fridge (this may not include the special fridge in a designated nursing room). Accidents happen, people could complain or throw it out, or you could forget your milk at work/school. You can get a personal office fridge if you have the space available to you.

When at home, do not store your milk in the door of the refrigerator or freezer. This will provide protection from changing temperatures. If you accidently leave your milk out overnight, it may still be safe to use the next day. Smell or taste the milk if you are unsure of its freshness. If the milk is not fresh or has sat out too long, you can use it for other nonedible milk products or a milk bath.

Freshly Expressed Breastmilk Storage Guidelines

Storage Location	Temperature	Time (Recommended)
Room Temp	66–75°F / 19–22°C	4–6 hours
Cooler Bag with Ice Block	59°F / 15°C	Up to 24 hours
Refrigerator	32–39°F / 0–4°C	5–7 days
Freezer (attached to fridge)	32°F / 0°C	3–4 months
Freezer (deep/chest)	0°F / -19°C	6–12 months

Thawed/ Previously Frozen Breastmilk Storage Guidelines

Storage Location	Temperature	Time (Recommended)
Room Temp	66–75°F / 19–22°C	1–2 hours
Cooler Bag with Ice Block	59°F / 15°C	Up to 24 hours
Refrigerator	32–39°F / 0–4°C	Up to 24 hours
Freezer (attached to fridge)	32°F / 0°C	Never refreeze
Freezer (deep/chest)	0°F / -19°C	Never refreeze

Partially thawed milk with ice crystals can still be considered frozen and is typically safe to refreeze. You can thaw breastmilk by holding it under running warm water, putting it in the refrigerator overnight, or by placing it in a bowl of warm water.

What if I don't have enough time to pump?

According to the law, a reasonable amount of time is allowed to a breastfeeding mother for the purposes of expressing milk for up to one year. (FYI: Your job does not need to know exactly how old your baby is for you to be able to pump. This is for those who may have returned to work later and still need to pump.) "A reasonable amount of time" is debatable, and you do not have to be paid for your time spent pumping. For the sake of argument, we will say "reasonable" is thirty minutes. That may not feel like enough time, but it is the goal we will try to meet based on the "reasonable" amount of time allotted to working mothers in many workplaces in the USA.

Maximize your pump time by:

- Having your parts clean and together
- Going straight to your pumping station/area
- Looking at pictures of your baby and/or listening to a baby crying or laughing
- Massaging the breasts

- Pumping for twenty consecutive minutes only! A double pump will make this quicker and easier, although this can be done with a single pump as well.
- Putting your used parts in the cooler bag with your expressed milk.

Keep sanitizer and cleanup wipes in your cooler bag as well. I suggest a natural cleanser for the start and end of your pump session. If you need more time because you have to walk a distance to the nursing room or because you feel the time allotted is not sufficient, ask for other accommodations in writing. If you have enough privacy, you could even express milk at your desk.

If you are an exclusive pumper, i.e., someone who has chosen to pump without latching, you can expect to produce twenty-four to thirty-six ounces in a twenty-four-hour period. The average baby eats about nineteen to thirty ounces daily. This is normal and nothing to worry about. Average breastmilk output is a half-ounce to four ounces for both breasts combined. Exclusively pumping will yield closer to two to four ounces per pump session. Only two to four ounces is needed to equal a normal feeding. Some women will have to pump two to three times to get enough for one feeding.

This is a sample chart of what a normal pumping and feeding schedule can look like with a minimum of eight pump sessions in a twenty-four-hour period. The bottles in this example are for every three hours, so I made them three ounces. I highly recommend bottles be made in two-ounce increments. This chart is for visual aid purposes.

Per Pump Session (Min. 8 sessions)	Per Bottle Feeding (Every 3 hours)	Baby Intake Per Feeding Session (Every 3 hours)
5 a.m. / 4 ounces	3 ounces	5 a.m. / 3 ounces
8 a.m. / 3.5 ounces	3 ounces	8 a.m. / 2.5 ounces
11 a.m. / 1.5 ounces	3 ounces	11 a.m. / 1.5 ounces
2 p.m. / 1.5 ounces	3 ounces	2 p.m. / 2.5 ounces
5 p.m. / 2 ounces	3 ounces	5 p.m. / 2 ounces
8 p.m. / 3 ounces	3 ounces	8 p.m. / 3 ounces
11 p.m. / 2.5 ounces	3 ounces	11 p.m. / 4 ounces
2 a.m. / 3 ounces	3 ounces	2 a.m. / 1.5 ounces
Total (in ounces): 21	Total: 24	Total: 20

This is a sample chart of what a normal pumping and feeding schedule can look like with twelve pump sessions in a twenty-four-hour period.

Per Pump Session (12 sessions)	Per Bottle Feeding (Every 2 hours)	Baby Intake Per Feeding Session (Every 2 hours)
5 a.m. / 3 ounces	2 ounces	5 a.m. / 2 ounces
7 a.m. / 3.5 ounces	2 ounces	7 a.m. / 3 ounces
9 a.m. / 2.5 ounces	2 ounces	9 a.m. / 2 ounces
11 a.m. / 1.5 ounces	2 ounces	11 a.m. / 2 ounces
1 p.m. / 4 ounces	2 ounces	1 p.m. / 1.5 ounces
3 p.m. / 2 ounces	2 ounces	3 p.m. / 1 ounce
5 p.m. / 1.5 ounces	2 ounces	5 p.m. / 1.5 ounces
7 p.m. / 2.5 ounce	2 ounces	7 p.m. / 1.5 ounce
9 p.m. / 2 ounces	2 ounces	9 p.m. / 2 ounces
11 p.m. / 1.5 ounces	2 ounces	11 p.m. / 3 ounces
1 a.m. / 2.5 ounces	2 ounces	1 a.m. / 1.5 ounces
3 a.m. / 3 ounces	2 ounces	3 a.m. / 3 ounces
Total (in ounces): 26.5	Total: 24	Total: 24

When preparing bottles, make two-ounce servings, label, and date them. If the baby is being sent to daycare or is left with a caregiver, you want to take special care in labeling each bottle with your child's name, the time for feeding, and the date. Make sure everyone practices pace feeding. Pace feeding is a method of bottle feeding that allows the baby to be more in control of the flow, the same way they are at the breasts. This practice is to avoid overfeeding the baby and wasting a large amount of milk, as some centers require leftover milk to be tossed after feedings.

How to Pace Feed:

- Size 0 or preemie nipples only. Your baby will never need a bigger hole or faster flow.
- Baby should always be sitting in an upright position.
- Bottle should be held horizontally.
- After twenty to thirty seconds, the bottle should be tipped downward to allow the milk to flow back into the bottle and out of the nipple. This gives baby a break and prevents overfeeding.
- Feeding should last ten to twenty minutes to mimic a "normal" feeding.
- Do not force your baby to finish the bottle if they are done eating. If they finish the bottle

and are still showing signs of hunger, switch arms and offer the second two-ounce bottle.

- Baby may not finish every bottle. Store the left-overs in the fridge and offer it first at the next feeding or use for other milk products.

During a growth spurt, your baby may begin to eat more frequently. You can signal your body to make more milk by power pumping to mimic cluster feeding. Power pumping using a double electric pump looks like this:

- Pump for twenty minutes, ten-minute pause, pump for ten minutes, ten-minute pause, pump for ten minutes, stop.
- The general recommendation is to repeat this up to three times a day.
- Repeat for three days, five maximum.

This can be done with a single electric and manual pump as well. Pump each side for an allotted time and move from one breast to the other for an hour. The goal is to achieve multiple letdowns to simulate cluster feeding.

- Pump for fifteen minutes on the right, pump for fifteen minutes on the left, pump for ten minutes on the right, pump for ten minutes on the left, pump for ten minutes on the right, then stop.

Change your pump parts on time. Keeping your parts up to date will allow your pump to work at an optimal level. An inefficient pump can stop suctioning and removing milk properly. This will mimic a dip in supply but will actually be a result of nonfunctioning parts. Set reminders in your phone, mark dates on your calendar, or schedule the parts to be shipped out ahead of time to ensure you are always pumping with functioning parts. The rule of thumb is to change parts after every sixty to eighty sessions.

Here is a chart with a more detailed change schedule.

Pump Parts	Replacement Frequency
Valves	2–8 weeks
Membranes	2–8 weeks
Duckbill Valves	4–12 weeks
Backflow Protectors	3–6 months
Tubing	3–6 months
Flanges	Every 6 months (or as needed)
Connectors	Every 6 months (or as needed)
Milk Collection Bottles	When chipped, cracked, or leaking

Read the instruction manual for your specific brand and pump type for more accurate information.

Support or Lack Thereof

Your coworkers may not be happy about you taking breaks to pump. Although it is none of their business, it can weigh on you and cause you to second-guess your decision. Having support from family/friends, a doula, a breastfeeding buddy, or a peer group can help you stay confident in your choice.

Your significant other may want to feed the baby and join in on the bonding experience. If someone is pressuring you to pump or use formula for their benefit, remind them that feeding the baby is your job, and they can help in other ways, such as bathing the baby, changing diapers, babywearing while you nap or shower, doing skin-to-skin contact, and burping the baby after you have finished a feeding session.

Other family members may pressure you to use formula as well. This is not necessary at all. Do not allow them to make you feel anything but joy about your choice to give your baby the best food they can have, made special by you. Being confident in your decision is the best way to ward off negativity. Remove yourself from any conversation that involves your parenting choices where you did not specifically ask for advice.

Pumping While in the NICU

If you are pumping while in the NICU, the pumping/feeding chart examples shown in this chapter may not be applicable to your situation. If your baby has a low birth weight or is premature, their stomachs are too small and they're too young to accommodate the amounts listed in the charts. The rules for pumping and guidelines for safe storage still apply. Label your milk with the date and time. If you need bottles, bags, labels, and other materials, you can ask your NICU nurses or social worker if they can supply them for you.

Change your pump parts on time. Eat and sleep as well as you can. Pace feed if using a bottle, and at every opportunity, practice latching your baby to your breasts. I suggest latching babies before offering supplemental feeding via bottle. This will help them learn how to breastfeed from the breasts and minimize nipple confusion or preference.

CHAPTER 8

✦ ◆ ✦

Travel, Shipping, Donations, and Medication

There are a number of reasons you may find yourself away from your baby for longer than the average work-day. If you find yourself traveling for work, follow the guidelines set up for the exclusively pumping moms. Express your milk, label, date, and store it. If you will be away less than five days (this includes commute time), it is safe for you to refrigerate your milk without needing to freeze it. Place the milk in a cooler with ice blocks/bags to transport it home safely. Once home, remember to put the milk in the freezer or use it immediately. Refer to the charts in Chapter 7 for safe storage guidelines.

Military Moms

Military moms, thank you for your service and the sacrifices you make while serving. Many factors will determine how well you are able to meet your breastfeeding goals, such as your commute, deployment, the age of your baby, and the length of deferred deployment.

Mom2Mom Global has a list of military policies for each branch, resources for lactation spaces, and insurance information. I found this to be one of the best online resources for military moms. Additionally, *Breastfeeding in Combat Boots: A Survival Guide to Successful Breastfeeding While Serving in the Military* is both a book and organization that helps support breastfeeding military women. They have an Instagram account that has uniform compliant, breastfeeding-friendly shirts and more helpful information.

Remember, the federal law for breastfeeding mothers also applies to the military. You do not have to end your breastfeeding journey if you and your baby are not ready.

Commuting by Car or Bus

You have more control in this scenario than others. Follow the safe storage guidelines and keep a close eye on your milk storage container when using public transportation. When properly stored, your milk should be fine during travel. Do not leave your milk in a rental car or a rideshare. Always have an eye on your milk and your breast pump when traveling in a shared vehicle.

When using public transportation with your baby, my suggestion is to babywear. This will keep your baby as close to you as possible for safety, comfort, and ease of breastfeeding. If you are driving or a passenger in a car, you will need to pull over to a safe destination before feeding your baby. Do not breastfeed while the car is in motion and never dangle over the child's car seat to feed them while the car is motion. This could result in life-threatening injuries for both you and your baby.

Traveling by Plane

The information I have regarding plane travel is for moms in the USA who are flying domestically. I cannot speak to the policies set by other countries when entering or exiting. These are the regulations set by the Transportation Security Administration (TSA).

- Breastmilk is permitted through security check-points. Remove the milk from your bag to be screened.

- There is no limit to the amount of breastmilk you can bring. "Reasonable quantities" are recommended.

- The TSA screens liquids by X-ray but may test breastmilk separately. Furthermore, the Food and Drug Administration (FDA) says there are no adverse effects from consuming food that has been screened by X-ray.

- A child does not need to be present for you to travel with your milk.

- Ice, ice blocks, and freezer packs are permitted to keep your milk cold.

- Dry ice is also permitted. The Federal Aviation Administration (FAA) limits you to five-and-a-half pounds of dry ice that is properly packaged, well-ventilated, and marked. Airline approval is required.

Print off the rules and regulations from the TSA website, have your milk in a separate bag or removed from your carry-on, and call ahead of time for peace of mind. If you are traveling internationally, please research the rules and regulations for transporting breastmilk for that country.

When traveling with your baby, it is best to nurse or give a bottle during takeoff and landing. This can help your baby stay calm during the transition and reduces the ear pain associated with the change in air pressure. Babywearing can help with discreet nursing and keep your hands free for ease of motion.

Shipping Breastmilk

Packaging Supplies:

- Sealable plastic bags
- Dry ice
- Thick Styrofoam cooler (for insulation and protection while traveling)

Shipping Supplies:

- Box/container that's bigger than the cooler
- Newspaper or packing paper
- Shipping labels
- Tape

How to Ship Breastmilk:

1. Express your milk and store it in bags or bottles.
2. Freeze it completely. Do not ship partially frozen milk.

3. Place your frozen milk into strong, sealable plastic bags. You can double the bags for extra security or wrap them in newspaper.

4. Add the bags to the Styrofoam cooler.

5. When handling dry ice, wear gloves. Put the dry ice on the bottom and sides of the cooler. Add a layer of your milk, then cover the breastmilk with more dry ice.

6. Any additional space in the cooler should be filled with newspaper or packing paper. This will prevent your milk from shifting during transport while also providing extra insulation.

7. Seal your package with tape. Vent the package to allow the vapors from the dry ice to escape. If not properly vented, your package can expand and possibly become damaged.

8. Place your sealed and vented cooler in a shipping container or box. Fill in the extra spaces with newspaper or packing paper, then seal the box.

9. Label your package and take it to a shipping center. Inform the associate you are shipping dry ice and human milk for proper storage and labeling. You should also call beforehand to verify they will accept dry ice packages.

10. Plan ahead to make sure your package arrives at the destination on time. Weekends and holidays

may result in delays, so please consider this before shipping during these times.

When packaged correctly, milk should remain frozen for overnight shipping up to two days.

Resources for Shipping

FedEx and UPS are recommended over USPS for shipping and tracking. ShipNEX is recommended for international shipping. Milk Expressed and LifeCare have partnered to provide breastmilk shipping for mothers. Milk Stork is another company that aims to make shipping breastmilk more convenient.

Donations

Donating milk or receiving milk donations can happen through milk banks, hospitals, organizations, and peer-to-peer resources. Lives can be saved by donating extra breastmilk. Any breastmilk contribution will have a big impact, as a premature infant can only eat a small amount per feeding but needs every drop. Donated milk can also benefit moms who have to be temporarily removed from their child or who have to temporarily stop breastfeeding for treatments that are not compatible with breastfeeding.

If you need donated breastmilk, you can join one of

the many online and social media groups, local groups, organizations, or milk banks in your area to receive milk. Use your discretion when contacting a mom directly for donated milk. Ask questions and use quantifiers before accepting the milk, such as plant-based, no medicine, no tobacco, no dairy, etc. This will help ensure the milk you receive will not upset your baby's tummy.

If you need to ship your donated milk, please refer to the shipping section in this chapter for details regarding safe shipping guidelines. Milk donations are a great resource, but do not feel forced to donate because you are breastfeeding. It can be an added pressure on a breastfeeding woman, and you are not obligated to donate.

Medication

Always consult your healthcare provider before starting or stopping any prescription medications. It is not uncommon for your doctor to be misinformed about the effect medications may have on the breastfeeding relationship. This can result in them suggesting that a mother pump and dump (which should never be done), stop breastfeeding for a few hours/days, or quit breastfeeding altogether to take the medication or treatment prescribed. Before following their directions, please do some research yourself, as most medications are compatible with breastfeeding.

Talking to an IBCLC or lactation consultant will yield information that is more helpful for your breastfeeding journey than the information most doctors will give you. This is because they study human lactation and have worked with a number of women and professionals, so they are better equipped to serve you. If you have more questions or are receiving conflicting information, please consult a lactation specialist about your doctor's and pharmaceutical company's opinions.

You can refer to the following lists of websites, apps, books, and call centers for any information you may need regarding medications' potential effects on the quality of your breastmilk.

Websites

- infantrisk.com
- toxnet.nlm.nih.gov/newtoxnet/lactmed.htm
- kellymom.com/hot-topics/med-risks/
- cdc.gov/breastfeeding

Apps (iPhone and Android)

- MommyMeds
- InfantRisk

Books

- *Medications and Mothers' Milk* by Thomas Hale, R.Ph, Ph.D

Call Centers

- The InfantRisk Center (1 806-352-2519) USA
- Drugs in Breastmilk (0844 412 4665) UK

CHAPTER 9

Nutrition and Self-Care

Keeping yourself healthy while breastfeeding is important. Eat well, stay hydrated, and take prenatal or postnatal vitamins to reduce your chances of becoming dehydrated and malnourished. As one cannot pour from an empty cup, it is imperative you eat and drink while nursing to replenish what your body takes from you to make nature's most perfect food.

While you are breastfeeding, your body will burn between three hundred and five hundred calories every day. Many women experience weight loss during their time nursing; on the other hand, some either don't have that experience or the opposite happens. To avoid dropping too many pounds, eat regularly and eat enough. If you want to avoid excessive weight gain, monitor your snacking. Sugary, high-calorie drinks and snacks can be replaced with water and fruit.

I cannot emphasize how important it is that you eat enough. Often, you will find yourself too tired to move, let alone eat. This is when being prepared will come in handy. Meal prepping once a week so you don't have to cook daily will be a great benefit to you and your family in the long run. Making easy-to-grab and no-heat options is one way to up your chances of eating a balanced meal. Making sandwiches, salads, casseroles, and smoothies are all quick and convenient food options. During your postpartum period, you will want to eat warm and hot foods for healing, so consider heating these foods in a microwave, a timer-set toaster oven, or any cooking device with an automatic shutoff mechanism. When you are tired, it is best to not attempt to cook. If you can manage, try to save oven-heated meals and non-cooked foods for a partner or family member. If you can't heat them quickly without risking falling asleep, do not risk it. Safety first.

Packing a snack box for your room is also a good idea—nuts, seeds (pumpkin, chia, flax, hemp), trail mix, chips, crackers, fruit (fresh or dried), nut butters, premade sandwiches (wrapped or in a container), hot soup or drinks in a thermos, water, and anything else you deem acceptable as snacks. These snacks are less for "health" and more for filling the tired mom's need to eat when she's too exhausted to make it to the kitchen. The goal is to eat as well as you are able to eat.

What you eat does not determine your supply output. Eat what you like, but remember that you need to be replacing essential vitamins and minerals for your optimal health. Common issues associated with essential nutrient deficiencies include tooth decay and cavities, hair loss and thinning (not to be confused with the normal postpartum shedding that occurs around four to seven months postpartum), weight loss, dull skin, memory issues, and fatigue. These are avoidable issues.

Breastfeeding is not the time to go on a diet, fast, detox, or calorie restrict. Doing so could introduce impurities into your milk. That is not to say you can't try new foods, transition to a plant-based diet, or remove certain foods from your diet. Just be aware of the effect doing so will have on you and your overall health.

Drink when you are thirsty. Do not drink "X amount of water a day" because you heard it would boost your milk supply. It won't work. Milk is made from your blood, not your gut. Drink enough to stay hydrated and quench your thirst.

Take care of yourself. Birthing a human life is a marvelous feat, and marvelous things need to be put back into you for you to function at your best. Focus on simple self-care tasks so you can nurture the garden that feeds your little one. Fifteen minutes can make all the difference in your day-to-day mothering activities. Spend some time alone bathing, brushing your teeth, moisturizing your hair, oiling your edges (postpartum shedding comes for us all), using good butters on your skin, getting fresh air, not cleaning (unless this relaxes you), lying naked in your bed, having a quickie with your partner (protect yourself from a future pregnancy if that is not on your mind right now), reading a new book, or meditating.

Nutrition for Babies

Babies' primary source of nutrition for the first year of life should be breastmilk or formula. After the age of one, your baby will not require a milk substitute if you choose to stop breastfeeding. No food should be given to a baby before the age of six months. Only start introducing foods to your baby if they are showing signs of readiness and are older than six months.

Signs of Readiness:

- Baby can sit up well without support.
- Baby has lost the tongue-thrusting reflex.
- Baby is willing to chew food and doesn't automatically push it out of their mouth.

- Baby has developed or is developing a pincer grasp.
- Baby can participate in meal time by picking up food and putting it into their own mouth.

If your baby is showing all the signs of readiness, then baby-led weaning is a great method for introducing solids to your little one. It is recommended by the WHO that babies be exclusively breastfed for the first six months of life, then with complimentary foods for two years. Some choose to breastfeed longer than two years. Breastfeeding should always be prioritized over any other food for the first year of life.

CHAPTER 10

✦ ◆ ✦

Taboo Topics and Questions

What do I need to eat to have the best breastmilk?

Eat what you would normally eat to stay healthy. Breastmilk is perfect and will be just right without much effort on your part. What you eat is for you! Eat well to replace the vitamins and nutrients your body uses for your milk. Drink to quench your thirst. Continue to take your prenatal vitamins or a breastfeeding-friendly postnatal supplement. Don't diet, fast, or cleanse while nursing because doing so could pass impurities from your breastmilk to your baby. Most of what you eat should not have a negative effect on your milk.

Mint, foods with decongestant properties, and some herbs, like fenugreek, can reduce your milk supply by a little or completely dry you up. Be careful with mother's milk teas, cookies, and other foods claiming to support milk production without researching and talking to an IBCLC. I do not recommend any product that claims to have milk-boosting properties.

Dairy can affect baby's digestion due to allergies or an intolerance. Reducing or removing all dairy from your diet will improve these issues, but not overnight. Give yourself and baby three to six weeks to adjust to the changes you have made before you begin to think it is not working. Dairy is in many types of packaged foods, so read labels carefully. It can take up to eight weeks for dairy to fully leave your system without a detox (which is not recommended while breastfeeding). I recommend waiting six weeks to see an improvement.

Words that mean dairy on food labels include:

- Butter
- Buttermilk
- Casein, Casein Hydrolysate, and Caseinates
- Cheese
- Cottage Cheese
- Cream
- Curds

- Diacetyl
- Ghee
- Lactalbumin
- Lactoferrin
- Lactose and Lactulose
- Milk
- Recaldent
- Sour Cream
- Whey
- Yogurt

My baby has gas. What can I do?

Babies grunt a lot. It is normal for them to make a lot of grunting sounds when they are young. This is not an indication that they are in pain or gassy. Also, breastmilk is easily digested. Their digestive system is working almost as soon as the milk touches the belly, which could be the cause of their grunting.

Symptoms of Gassiness:

- Arching the back and pulling legs up
- Swollen-looking or pushed out stomach
- Excessive burping or flatulence

Gas symptoms can be relieved using bicycle legs, tummy time, and burping the baby more often during

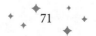

and after feeding sessions. *Do not* give your baby anything other than breastmilk to treat gas. This includes but is not limited to:

- Gripe water
- Gas drops
- Karo syrup
- Natural remedies

Breastmilk has everything your baby needs, and nothing else should be given to them to "treat" gas. These are outdated methods, and I do not recommend them, as they could cause harm to the baby's digestive system.

Can I drink alcohol?

Yes. Have a drink, sis. Don't get party-girl wasted and don't dump your milk. As long as you are safe to drive, you are still safe to nurse your little one. If you are slurring your words, stumbling, or unable to keep your eyes open, you are likely too drunk to breastfeed. If you are unsure about serving your baby milk with even a trace amount of alcohol in it, then pump and use the milk for a milk bath. Not drinking is the safest option while breastfeeding, but the occasional drink is OK. Do not bed-share with your baby while drinking or under the influence.

The Dietary Guidelines for Americans defines a standard "drink" as:

- 12 ounces of 5% beer
- 8 ounces of 7% malt liquor
- 5 ounces of 12% wine
- 1.5 ounces of 40% (80 proof) liquor

All of these drinks contain the same amount, fourteen grams or 0.6 ounces, of pure alcohol.

Over time, excessive alcohol consumption can lead to shortened breastfeeding duration due to decreased milk production. Excessive alcohol consumption while breastfeeding could also affect the infant's sleep patterns and early development.

Can I use cannabis?

This is a tricky question. Yes, you can smoke weed while breastfeeding, but treat the secondhand smoke the same as you would cigarette smoke. The body naturally produces cannabinoids and very few would pass through to your breastmilk from smoking; however, you want to be safe and responsible while using cannabis and breastfeeding, as it can alter your mood and state of mind. If you are able to perform normal daily activities and properly care for your baby, then you may be OK. I also do not recommend mothers use tobacco products for smoking. Instead, use glass or hemp paper. There are other methods of ingesting cannabis as well. Do not bed-share while under the influence of cannabis products.

Some short-term research has suggested a few children exposed to mothers who smoked while breastfeeding had lower cognitive functions and poor memory in comparison to their peers. The research may not account for home and lifestyle, diet, schooling, or other factors outside of marijuana use (not including the amount or preparation). Other research suggests a delay in motor functions but not cognitive or intellectual functions. Sources on this topic are cited in the bibliography so you can do your own research and make an informed decision for you and your family. CBD oil and tinctures could be a solution for you if you are against pharmaceuticals. CBD, cannabis, and weed are names for the same hemp plant but speak to different properties and uses.

Can I get a tattoo?

No, or at least you shouldn't. Technically, a tattoo artist could still tattoo you if you want one, but it is not recommended due to the risk of infection.

Is it safe to breastfeed with nipple piercings and/or post-breast reduction or enlargement?

You can still breastfeed if you have had your breasts augmented. Piercings should be removed during pregnancy and while breastfeeding. The hole for the piercing may close if it's not fully healed. If the hole is healed, you can expect milk to flow or leak from the area during a letdown or before a feeding. You should not get any piercings, nipple or otherwise, while breastfeeding due to risk of infection.

There are different types of breast reductions and enlargements, and your ability to breastfeed will be impacted by the type of incision and closure you had. The majority of women do not see a decrease in milk production or flow. Check with an IBCLC to discuss your personal circumstances. Implants generally have no effect on a woman's ability to breastfeed.

What if my child's father/guardian and I are no longer partners or cohabitating?

Mediation. Establish a visitation schedule that allows you to have primary care of the baby so breastfeeding can be established before overnight visits take place. As you will still have to pump throughout the night while baby is away, it is easier to keep baby with you. Compile all the breastfeeding evidence that supports your decision to breastfeed, research your local law and the federal laws, consult a breastfeeding-friendly and supportive doctor, and hire a lawyer if needed. My advice is to try to keep this out of court if at all possible. The courts do not have your family's best interest at heart, and they are going to do what they think is "fair."

How will breastfeeding affect my sex life/sex drive?

For some women, breastfeeding can decrease sex drive and vaginal lubrication. For others, sex drive will increase. It depends on the woman, her birth experience, how important her breasts are during sex and foreplay, and other factors like her quality of sleep and self-care.

Some spouses can feel jaded by a breastfeeding mom. This is not uncommon. Their attitude stems from them feeling that the baby is getting all the love and affection, while they are being excluded from the family bonding experience. Others may be very aroused by leaking breasts and, for some, even the taste of breastmilk, which is normal. Communicate openly about what you are comfortable with, and don't put too much pressure on your breasts. Most men learned to associate breasts with sex but not breastfeeding a child. In western cultures, this is quite common and needs to be discussed honestly. Breasts are for nurturing the young life you've created together, but they can also be used during lovemaking.

Can breastfeeding cause me to be aroused?

Some women have experienced arousal while breastfeeding. It is normal, but many women still feel a great deal of guilt about it. No one should feel guilty about feeling a sense of arousal. The reaction is completely involuntary.

Sexual Trauma

Past sexual trauma can make it hard to breastfeed a baby. There are books and blogs dedicated to this subject matter, and these should be read by anyone who desires to breastfeed and has experienced trauma related to sex, birth, or any form of physical violence that may prevent them from doing so uninhibited.

CHAPTER 11

✦ ◆ ✦

Breastfeeding Stories

Story One:

I became a mother during my senior year of high school, right before I was scheduled to go off to college. My intention throughout my pregnancy was to breastfeed for at least a year, as my mother had breastfed me. I spoke to my OB-GYN, nurses, my mother, teachers, and pediatrician about my desire to breastfeed my child, and not one of them gave me a book, mentioned a class, suggested a group, or sat me down to give me the details I would need to succeed on my journey. I didn't even know where to start and had no clue I would need to do research.

Once my son was born, I waited in my hospital room for the nurses to bring him from the nursery when they thought he was ready to be fed. I assumed breastfeeding would be easy because it was instinctual, and if I needed help, people would support me. This was not the case. My nurses became agitated at my lack of skill and gave my son a bottle of formula and said we would try again later. This upset me, but I was tired and needed to rest, so I sat back against my support pillow and went to sleep. The next feeding came quickly, and I awoke to a nurse bringing my son back in my room with a pacifier in his mouth. This time, I requested that he not be removed from my room, as I wanted to learn to breastfeed and not use formula. The nurses sent a lactation consultant into my room to help. This woman did not help me at all. She was forceful, mean, and made me feel less than for not being able to use her methods on the first try.

At that point, I asked for a breast pump and said I would exclusively pump for my son to get the breast-milk I so desperately wanted him to have. I barely got an ounce of milk on my first try. The pump was painful because my breasts were tender. No one told me this was normal and that I should not worry. No one gave me words of encouragement or helpful suggestions on how to make things easier for me, and I felt like I had lost that battle.

Home was not any better. My mother decided that, because I made a baby, I should be solely responsible for caring for him. I was still finishing high school and college courses, preparing to graduate, and learning how to breastfeed/exclusively pump three days postpartum, and now, I was being made to prepare my own food and clean during the times I should have been sleeping. To say I was exhausted would be a gross understatement. I was pumping barely six times a day and honestly did not know any better. I thought as long as I was getting milk for him to drink, it did not matter how frequently I expressed my milk.

I continued on this way for two months. Every day, my mom suggested I stop because she thought I was too tired, wasn't eating enough, my body was withering away, blah, blah, blah. Day in and day out, I listened to her reminders that I was not doing well on my journey. At my son's second doctor's appointment, the pediatrician wanted to know if I was still breastfeeding, to which I answered, "Yes." He asked how much my son was eating and all the relevant questions I was too tired to answer correctly. When I asked him about my son spitting up frequently, he suggested I give my little one formula. Why? Because formula was heavier than breastmilk, and he would keep it down better. This began the end of my breastfeeding journey. We only made it four months before I could no longer take my mother's words, the doctor's "help," and the exhausting days that led to insomnia.

Story Two:

I was in my twenties when I gave birth to my second child. Breastfeeding had been on my mind heavily, and I requested that a nurse or LC come to my home to help me. They both came and were incredibly helpful, but I still underestimated how hard breastfeeding could be without proper preparation. My son latched perfectly on my right breast and fed well. His latch on my left breast was painful, and I cringed at the thought of having him on that side. The pain caused me to begin to pump just over a week into my journey. Doing this resulted in a massive oversupply, which I was happy to have because of my previous experience. An oversupply is not a positive and is just as, if not more, detrimental as a low supply from not expressing milk. I started to stock the freezer with my surplus of milk. My breasts were always engorged, and I had no idea the kind of issues my obsession would lead me to on that road.

During a snowstorm, the power went out. My entire freezer stash, totaling roughly sixty ounces or more, thawed out while I was away from home. I returned to find my stash ruined. This broke my heart. Luckily, some of my milk was being stored with the babysitter, and I did not need to replace those feedings to return to work.

We made it roughly six to seven months exclusively breastfeeding before food was introduced. My son really loved eating and preferred to take his milk about four times a day before a meal and then eat the rest of the time, with a few nursing sessions on the nights he didn't sleep. We did this until he was a year old before we switched him to non-dairy milk, and I officially stopped breastfeeding.

Story Three:

My third son was born, and I was determined to make it work this time. Everything was going well until I got my first clogged duct. The pain was unbelievable, and I called upon my husband to let me dangle feed him. He was more than happy to help me relieve the pain. After that situation was handled, the little one and I got thrush. My breasts were not ready for the fungal outbreak, but I was mentally prepared to handle anything. We got the medicine, and the treatment worked well for both of us.

Well, would you believe that more problems arose during this experience? Barely a month later, I was pumping in preparation to leave the baby with my husband when I placed the pump to my breast and heard a sound like paper tearing then felt the pain across my areola and nipple. I immediately shut the pump off and slowly removed it from my chest. To my horror, I saw blood. I did not panic. I swiftly opened the bottle to retrieve the drops of expressed milk and began coating the area with it. You may have already guessed that I tore my nipple. This happened as a result of the pump setting being up too high (whether it was speed or pressure I do not remember).

The injury healed, but during that time, I still needed to express milk from that breast. I used a combination of a warm cloth, massage techniques, and hand-expressing about seven to nine times a day for the next week to release milk. My areola was constantly coated with my milk and coconut oil to promote healing.

After all of those mishaps and misfortunes, I was still able to continue breastfeeding for almost a year. We began to supplement with formula due to misinformation from the pediatrician about frequent feedings and sleep, but overall, I was proud of myself.

Story Four:

Now armed with more knowledge on what not to do while breastfeeding, I wanted to know what I needed to do to succeed. I joined a breastfeeding group headed by professionals who worked as nurses, LCs, IBCLCs, and doctors. This group saved me from failure and likely saved my twins' lives.

In the summer of 2018, my husband and I were told we were expecting twins. This news came as a pleasant shock. We both researched twin pregnancy, cloth diapers, NICUs in the state, and homebirth for multiples. Our birth team consisted of our doula, midwife, midwife in training, and a colleague of hers for additional support. We met with OB-GYNs and selected a supportive and thoughtful doctor to be our backup. As luck would have it, our OB-GYN was also a twin mom. Everything was going well, so I began to dive deep into breastfeeding education. I spent hours reading research, best practices, storage guidelines, and surfing through the breastfeeding group for other twin moms who succeeded on their breastfeeding journeys.

Our babies were born at thirty-two weeks via emergency cesarean and were taken away to the NICU forty-five minutes away. I will not go into details here about the hardships I faced post-cesarean birth, but I have written a blog post detailing the events on my website (onlyblackstarsinthesky.org) titled "In Honor of Black Maternal Health Week."

I left the hospital forty-eight hours post-surgery to head over to the NICU to see my newborns. They were in isolates to keep them warm and were just over four pounds. I told my nurses I would be exclusively breastfeeding, and I was happy to see how swiftly they moved to get me a chair, a breast pump (both manual and electric), bottles, and labels. They provided me with so many amenities to ensure my success that it brought me to tears. I was so happy I had done all the research to find a breastfeeding-friendly hospital with a supportive staff. Many of the staff members were breastfeeding mothers themselves, so this opened up a great dialogue.

Doctors came around to make suggestions on how to best help the babies gain weight. The babies were both gaining weight at a steady pace and had no other health concerns, so I was confused when the conversation was brought up. Even with the feeding tubes, the babies were able to latch, although most of their feedings were via the feeding tube. The doctor raised concerns that I would not be able to continue breastfeeding when I was home with the twins outside of the hospital setting. I assured them I was well-informed of what was to come and had prepared for this as much as I could. I was confident in my ability to continue breastfeeding outside of the hospital setting. This was not good enough for them.

In the days that followed, I was given books, research, videos, and more information than I could ever ask for, and I was pleased. I read through most of the information, watched the videos, and consulted with them again about my decision to exclusively breast-feed my children. This time, they set up a meeting with about eight professionals, none of whom were an LC or IBCLC, to try to talk me into bottle-feeding my little ones. I was flabbergasted. After all the research they had given me on breastfeeding, I felt they had not read it themselves. Calmly, I suggested they go through their own research before sitting down with me again because nothing I read or watched suggested that pree-mies would be at a disadvantage if they were not fed via bottle. I mentioned how babies could be fed via spoon, syringe, dropper, or cup and that an artificial nipple was not needed for success or health.

This conversation did not go over well, and while they all left the room congratulating themselves on having convinced me of their way, I felt betrayed by the very people who were so compassionate just days before. I could not understand why I was being told I would not succeed when I had been producing milk, keeping my babies fed, both babies were healthy, and I demonstrated I was knowledgeable about breastfeed-ing. To leave the hospital with my children, I had to compromise on using the bottle so the doctors could see just how much the babies were ingesting per feed-ing. This became another task, as I had to religiously document every feeding and diaper output and time for two newborns.

After thirty days in the NICU, we were finally discharged. A weight was lifted off of my shoulders, and I felt I could conquer the world. My babies latched well, and I continued to supplement with one-ounce bottles of my own milk after every feeding. As I grew tired of the manual breast pump, I switched over to the silicone milk catcher that acted as a pseudo pump. This continued on for about five months, then the little ones did not need the expressed milk anymore. We breastfed together for twenty-two months before I became pregnant with another child and my milk production slowed.

Final Thoughts

I started my breastfeeding journey as a young mother who had no idea what breastfeeding really meant. My hopes for success were outweighed by misinformation, formula suggestions, and constant criticism. I spent many years making mistakes, regretting past decisions, and wishing I had the information available to me when I needed it the most. After many years of reading research, following professionals, and learning firsthand how much work goes into a successful breastfeeding experience, I wrote this book. My goal was to create a comprehensive, easy-to-read guide to encourage mothers to continue breastfeeding and seek help before it's too late.

Now that I have successfully tandem nursed my twins through our time spent in the NICU up to their second birthday, I feel confident in my ability to share the education, research, tips, and tools I have stockpiled over the years. In my efforts to educate more women on breastfeeding, I founded Only Black Stars in the Sky, an organization to support birth workers, lactation experts, and families transitioning into parenthood. For more information about my work, you can visit my website at onlyblackstarsinthesky.org and my Instagram @onlyblackstarsinthesky for information regarding breastfeeding, natural parenting, and healthy living.

The best advice I can give to anyone would be to be cautious of whom you decide to share your breastfeeding goals with. Some may be supportive and encouraging, while others may attempt to dissuade you. This advice is not exclusive to family and friends. Even medical professionals can give bad advice, as breastfeeding is not commonly studied by doctors or they are mostly familiar with outdated information.

Please do not take my words to mean you cannot discuss your plans, joys, or all things breastfeeding with anyone at any point during your journey. You can and you should, as this will help normalize breastfeeding. My suggestion is to simply be aware of how people feel about mothers who choose to breastfeed before you open yourself up to potential scrutiny. I find this to be especially true for mothers who are preparing to breastfeed for the first time, young moms, parents of multiples, and women with disabilities.

Contact a professional for specific answers to your questions. Breastfeeding requires roughly 140 minutes a day, three hundred to five hundred calories burned, and consistent hydration. Breastfeeding is a sport! You can do this with proper education and training. Join the Breastfeeding Support Group for Black Moms on Facebook for continuous community support, education modules, and access to years of research and data from professionals. I wish you well on your breastfeeding journey, and if this book helped you in any way, consider gifting a copy to another mom.

Bibliography

Bonyata, Kelly. "Breastfeeding Your Newborn — What to Expect in the Early Weeks." Kellymom.com.

Cassidy, Dianne. "Emotional and Physical Trauma and Its Impact on Breastfeeding Mothers." *Clinics in Human Lactation* 14.

Centers for Disease Control and Prevention. cdc.gov/breastfeeding/breastfeeding-special-circumstances/vaccinations-medications-drugs/alcohol.html (Page last reviewed: January 24, 2018.)

Centers for Disease Control and Prevention. "Is It Safe for Mothers Who Use Marijuana to Breastfeed?" Cdc.gov. (Page last reviewed: January 24, 2018.)

Dietary Guidelines for Americans. *HHS Publication* 8, (2015-2020). health.gov/dietaryguidelines/2015/guidelines/appendix-9/

Drugs and Lactation Database. Bethesda, MD: National Library of Medicine (US) 2006, Cannabis.

Ghaheri, Bobby. "Tongue and Lip Tie FAQ." (October 2, 2014) drghaheri.squarespace.com/blog/2014/10/2/tongue-tie-and-lip-tie-faq.

Hale, Thomas Ph.D. "Dr. Thomas Hale on Coconut Oil and Breastmilk." (October 10, 2012) www.infantrisk.com/forum/forum/medications-and-breastfeeding-mothers/medications-and-mothers-milk/803-coconut-oil-on-breast.

Heise, Alla. "Before the Letdown: Dysphoric Milk Ejection Reflex and the Breastfeeding Mother." D-MER.org

International Code of Marketing of Breast-Milk Substitutes. World Health Organization 1981. who.int/nutrition/publications/code_english.pdf

Klingelhafer, Susan Kathleen. "Sexual Abuse and Breastfeeding." Vol. 23, no. 2 (May 2007): 194–197

Lexico (Powered by Oxford). Dictionary.com and Oxford University Press (OUP) 2020. www.lexico.com

MacDonald, Elizabeth. "The Golden Hour After Birth." *My Baby's Heartbeat Bear.* March 7, 2019.

Meier, Paula P., Engstrom, Janet L., Patel, Aloka L., Jegier, Briana J., and Bruns, Nicholas E. "Improving the Use of Human Milk During and After the NICU Stay." *Clinics in Perinatology* 37, no. 1 (March 2011): 217–245.

Nangia, Paul, Deorari, Sreenivas, Agarwal, and Chawla. "Topical Oil Application and Trans-Epidermal Water Loss in Preterm Very Low Birth Weight Infants—A Randomized Trial." *Journal of Tropical Pediatrics.* (December 2015) www.ncbi.nlm.nih.gov/pubmed/26338490?dopt=Abstract

National Center for Complementary and Integrative Health (NCCIH). nccih.nih.gov/health/colloidalsilver (Page last updated: April 2017.)

Neczypor, Jennifer L., Holley, Sharon L. "Providing Evidence-Based Care During the Golden Hour." Vol. 21, no. 6 (December 2017): 462–472.

Polomeno, Viola. "Sex and Breastfeeding: An Educational Perspective." *The Journal of Perinatal Education*, (Winter 1999).

Stuebe, Allison. "The Risks of Not Breastfeeding for Mothers and Infants." *Reviews in Obstetrics and Gynecology* 2, no. 4 (Fall 2009): 222–23. ncbi.nlm.nih.gov/pmc/articles/PMC2812877/

Sachs, Hari Cheryl and Committee on Drugs. "The Transfer of Drugs and Therapeutics Into Human Breast Milk: An Update on Selected Topics." *Official Journal of The American Academy of Pediatrics.* (September 2013) pediatrics.aappublications.org/content/132/3/e796

WIC Breastfeeding Support. U.S. Department of Agriculture. wicbreastfeeding.fns.usda.gov. (December 13, 2019.)

Wolf, Jacqueline H. "'Mercenary Hirelings' or 'A Great Blessing'?: Doctors' and Mothers' Conflicted Perceptions of Wet Nurses and the Ramifications for Infant Feeding in Chicago, 1871-1961." *Journal of Social History* 33, no. 1 (Autumn, 1999): 97-120. jstor.org/stable/3789462

Glossary

Areola – The dark circle of pigmentation around the nipple. Acts as a target for the baby to find their food source.

Baby-led weaning – A method of starting your baby on solids that bypasses purees and goes straight to finger foods.

Babywearing – The method of carrying a baby in a sling or wrapping a baby to be carried on the body.

Breastfeeding – The action of feeding a baby with milk made from the breast, including nursing from the breast, pumping, and feeding via bottle or another tool.

Breastmilk – Also known as mother's milk, breastmilk is the milk produced by the breasts of a female to feed a child. Milk is the primary source of nutrition for newborns before they are able to eat and digest other foods. Contains immunologic agents and other compounds that protect the baby against viruses, bacteria, and parasites.

Cluster feeding – The way your baby boosts your milk supply by nursing frequently, typically during a growth spurt.

Coconut oil (extra virgin) – Commonly called MCT oil. This oil is used in some NICUs to add fat into the diets of premature infants. Easily digested by all neonates and older children. Coconut oil has many benefits for the skin and body.

Colloidal silver – A solution with silver particles that has antiseptic properties. A traditional remedy that has been used for centuries to treat a variety of ailments, including pneumonia, skin rashes, sinus infections, flu, and more.

Colostrum – The first secretion from the mammary glands after giving birth, rich in antibodies. Also referred to as liquid gold.

Delayed cord clamping – Waiting before clamping or cutting the umbilical cord to allow more blood to transfer from the placenta to the baby.

Dysphoric Milk Ejection Reflex (D-MER) – An anomaly of the milk release mechanism in lactating women. A brief dysphoria just prior to letdown.

Engorgement – Swelling that occurs with increased blood flow and milk to your breasts in the first few days after giving birth to a baby. Can also occur when the breasts are painfully overfull with milk due to too much milk being produced, also known as an oversupply.

ENT – Ear, nose, and throat specialist/doctor.

Exclusive pumper/pumping – Moms who choose to bottle-feed their infants expressed breastmilk only.

Feeding on demand – The practice of feeding at the first sign of baby's hunger cues rather than on a set schedule.

Fenugreek – An herb used as a ground seed in capsule form or in a tea to increase milk production. Can have adverse effects by decreasing breastmilk production in some women.

Foremilk – Refers to milk at the beginning of a feeding.

Formula – Infant formula, baby formula, or just formula is a manufactured food designed and marketed to feed babies and infants under twelve months of age. It's usually prepared for bottle-feeding or cup-feeding from powder or liquid and is commonly made with cow's milk. Designed to be roughly based on human milk at one to three months postpartum.

Gentian violet – An antiseptic dye used to treat fungal infections of the skin, such as ringworm and athlete's foot. It also has weak antibacterial effects and may be used on minor cuts and scrapes to prevent infection.

Golden hour – The first sixty minutes after birth. This time is important to help baby transition from the womb to the outside world.

Hindmilk – Refers to milk at the end of a feeding.

Human Milk Fortifier (HMF) – An additive to breastmilk that provides additional calories and nutrition for premature infants. One is made from cow's milk, and the other is made from human milk that was donated by healthy nursing mothers.

International Board-Certified Lactation Consultant (IBCLC) – A healthcare professional who specializes in the clinical management of breastfeeding. IBCLCs are certified by the International Board of Lactation

Consultant Examiners, Inc. under the direction of the U.S. National Commission for Certifying Agencies.

Instruction manual – Please read the instruction manual to everything you use, especially your breast pump. Details on how to clean your breast pump and how to replace pump parts can be found in the instruction manual.

Jaundice – Newborn jaundice is very common and can occur when babies have a high level of bilirubin, a yellow pigment produced during the normal breakdown of red blood cells. Can be treated with breastmilk and indirect sunlight. Most babies will get better in one to two weeks without medical treatment.

Kangaroo care – A type of bonding that promotes skin-to-skin contact and babywearing to help stimulate feelings of closeness and well-being for both mother/ parents and baby.

Lactation consultant – A health professional who specializes in the clinical management of breastfeeding.

Lactoferrin – A protein present in human milk with iron-binding, antibacterial, antiviral, antiparasitic, catalytic, anti-cancer, and anti-allergic functions and properties.

Letdown reflex – An involuntary reflex during the period of time when a woman is breastfeeding which causes the milk to flow freely. This reflex can feel like tingling, pins and needles, achiness, or throbbing sensations. A forceful letdown can be painful and is often the result of an oversupply or overabundant milk production.

Lip tie – A tight frenulum (skin between the lip and the gums) that impedes breastfeeding.

Liquid gold – The nectar of life. Breastmilk at every stage from colostrum to mature milk. The living organism that will change to suit your baby's needs. It is food, drink, medicine, and love made by mothers everywhere.

Mastitis – Inflammation of the mammary gland in the breast due to a bacterial infection. Trapped milk in the breast is the main cause of mastitis.

Mature milk – Milk produced in as great a volume as transitional milk but is thinner and watery or even bluish in color. Often compared to skim milk.

MCT oil – A fat supplement that is easily absorbed by the skin and body. Added to the feedings of infants who need extra calories for weight gain. Medium-chain triglyceride. Extra virgin coconut oil.

Mother's milk teas – Herbal teas claiming to promote milk production for lactating mothers. Main ingredient is often fenugreek.

Neonates – Newborns or infants less than four weeks old.

Nipple confusion – An occurrence, also known as nipple preference, that happens when an artificial nipple, such as pacifiers and bottles, are offered too soon or before breastfeeding is properly established. Does not affect all babies.

Oversupply – When the breasts are producing an overabundance of milk. This can result in a forceful letdown that causes a baby to choke, gag, or be unsettled at the breasts. When left untreated, an oversupply can lead to other breast-related issues, such as mastitis.

Oxytocin – A hormone released by the pituitary gland that stimulates the ejection of milk into the ducts of the breasts and causes increased contraction of the uterus during labor. Also referred to as the love hormone.

Postpartum shedding – Hormonal hair loss due to the stage the hair enters during the postpartum period. Commonly associated with the loss of edges and thinning hair volume.

Power pumping – A method of pumping intended to mimic the cluster feeding and growth spurt phase of a breastfeeding baby that boosts milk production.

Prolactin – A hormone produced by the pituitary gland in the brain mainly used to help women produce milk after childbirth. Also known as PRL or lactogenic hormone.

Pump and dump – The term used to describe the act of expressing or pumping breastmilk then discarding or dumping it. This is an outdated concept and a waste of liquid gold.

Rooting – An involuntary, active sign of hunger evident as a baby moves the head around looking for a nipple to latch on to for feedings.

Skin to skin – Refers to the bare skin bodily contact between mother and child. Skin-to-skin contact can be made with any member of the family, but it is important that the mother establish this connection with the newborn to promote breastfeeding.

Supplemental feeds – Additional feedings given to a baby using the mother's expressed milk. Usually 0.5 to one-and-a-half ounces (partial but not a whole feeding).

Trans-Epidermal Water Loss (TEWL) – The amount of water that passively evaporates through skin. Used to characterize skin barrier function.

Tongue tie – A condition where the lingual frenulum (tissue connecting the tongue to the floor of the mouth) is short and tight, restricting tongue movement and breastfeeding ability.

Top-up trap – The top-up trap refers to the method of breastfeeding then overfeeding/supplementing with formula. This usually happens as a result of the mother or caregiver not being confident that the baby is full after consuming breastmilk. Doing this can result in a decreased milk supply due to milk not being removed or stimulated at the breasts. It can also cause the baby to be overfed, which will result in a stretched stomach.

Transitional milk – The creamy milk that follows colostrum. Typically seen around two to five days postpartum.

Two-shirt method – Refers to a method of discreetly breastfeeding by wearing a camisole or tank top underneath a loose-fitting shirt so one can then lift the shirt and pull down the camisole to breastfeed comfortably.

Vernix – The white, creamy-like substance your baby is coated in at birth. It is composed of water, protein, and lipids. Rub it into the baby's skin for health benefits, like protection against harmful bacteria and soft, smooth skin. It is commonly linked to the "new baby smell."

Wet nurse – A woman who breastfeeds and cares for another's child. These women are employed if the mother is unable or elects not to nurse the child herself. Wet-nursed children may be known as "milk siblings," and in some cultures, the families are linked by a special relationship of milk kinship.

Women, Infants, and Children (WIC) – The Special Supplemental Nutrition Program for Women, Infants, and Children is a federal assistance program of the Food and Nutrition Service of the United States Department of Agriculture for the health care and nutrition of low-income pregnant women, breastfeeding women, and children under the age of five.

Thank you for reading
The Melanated Milkyway Breastfeeding Guidebook
If you found this book resourseful,
please leave an online review.

KEEP IN TOUCH WITH SHAQUANNA

Website: www.onlyblackstarsinthesky.com
Instagram: @onlyblackstarsinthesky
Facebook: Quanni Thomas Covington
Twitter: @_onlyblackstars

Made in the USA
Columbia, SC
29 September 2020